EXAMEN

EXAMEN

POEMS

SUSAN SINK

lulu.com

ISBN 978-1-304-976062

Book design and layout by Kenji Liu
Cover photo by Susan Sink
Section illustrations by Oliver Smith

Source: *The Collected Poems of Stanley Kunitz,* (W. W. Norton and Co., Inc., 2002)

FOR KATHY BECKER AND DALE ELIZABETH SINK

Christ with me, Christ before me, Christ behind me,

Christ in me, Christ beneath me, Christ above me,

Christ on my right, Christ on my left,

Christ when I lie down, Christ when I sit down,

Christ in the heart of every person who thinks of me,

Christ in the mouth of every person who speaks of me,

Christ in the eye of every person who sees me,

Christ in the ear of everyone who hears me.

—PRAYER OF ST. PATRICK

Some words on "the Examen": St. Ignatius of Loyola, founder of the Jesuits, encouraged his community members to engage in a prayer practice of examining their consciences through an examination of their daily lives. His practice including asking questions and identifying moments where one was more centered on God's love and where one fell short. Over time, what is being observed and discerned has been reframed by spiritual writers and practitioners. Always it is a process of looking for God in daily life and the world in order to love others well. One reframing I like is to identify moments of consolation and desolation in the day. This is a collection of such moments.

CONTENTS

I

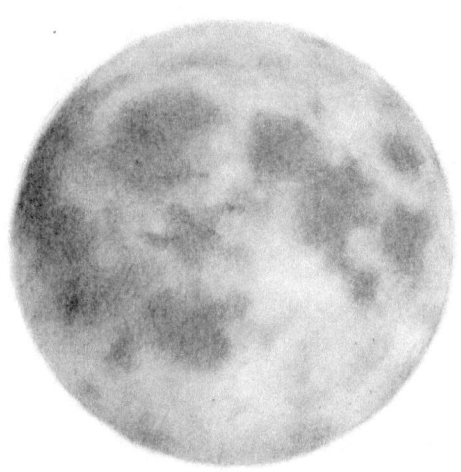

HOW LONG HAVE YOU BEEN A POET?

AFTER JAMES TATE'S FINAL POEM, "I SAT AT MY DESK AND
CONTEMPLATED ALL THAT I HAD ACCOMPLISHED THIS YEAR."

I've been a poet since twenty-six.
I won a big prize and everyone agreed
my work transcended the personal to the universal.
My best-selling first book was greeted with awe.

I've been a poet since I was ten.
I wrote fifty books of haiku that year
on my father's Royal typewriter.
The ribbon printed in red and black.

I wrote a famous poem about air pollution.
It hung on the classroom bulletin board.
My poem about litter was not as strong.
Less emotionally honest and somewhat trite.

I've been a poet since I was two.
My first poem went like this:
Ball
Moon
I recited it every chance I got.

I was a poet in my mother's womb,
tumbling around, eyes wide open,
everything red, then black, then red.
I was intricate. I was luminous.

I was a much better poet all those years
before my incarnation. Out there
spinning with the spheres,
singing our songs, shining our light.

Our light took centuries to reach earth.
By then, no one could translate.
Scientists worked in a binary code,
a language that disallowed metaphor.

God was impressed with our systems:
time, space, architecture, the silicon chip.
But our poetry, God thought, suffered.

WHEN WERE YOU HAPPIEST IN YOUR BODY?

I weigh the pleasure of a naked swim alone
in a deep glacial pool in Desolation Wilderness
against another, with my lover and the public
on a nude beach at Lake Tahoe, the Nevada side.
Clothed only in clear water, visible and light,
moving to a rock, I was not ashamed or scared.
In the deep dark cold of the lake, or warmed
against a granite shelf, I loved my body then.

Other moments, in yoga folding back to child's pose
feeling myself small and compact, or on one side,
full weight on my hand and stretched like a kite,
or when the strength I didn't know I had
lifted my whole body straight up in my first
stunned headstand shouting look at me, look at me.

WHEN WERE YOU HAPPIEST IN YOUR BODY? (II)

When I enter my own bathroom I see
the small square print of Degas' bather
and am astonished at my own body there,
the heaviness of belly and firm thighs
as she sits on her heels in the basin
and moves the towel along the flesh
inside her arm, a gesture with no reason
but the aesthetic value of her own gaze.
Sometimes I blush when I discover
myself there, it's true. Can one come this late
to the body, in middle age, and learn to accept
a simple touch one might name happiness?
Maybe happiness in my skin is still to come.
Let me learn it from your fingers and your tongue.

WHAT WAS THE DARKEST NIGHT?

It was in the woods in Saratoga Springs,
after a party with champagne and strawberries we took
a drawbridge to reach. It was so dark we could not see
the path, our own white tennis shoes, our hands before our faces.
We could see fireflies, though, a thousand fireflies, that gave
the dark a depth and width and height. No moon, no stars,
no light except those flashing, pulsing, love-lit tails
and the slow, languorous way they wove through the air.

Their flight was in our very blood. And though
it was a month of nightmares, dark revelations,
the month I learned I would not take my life
and how close I could come, I almost cried for joy
in that darkness. My laughter went up through the invisible trees,
like birdsong, like champagne, a flock of doves released.

WHAT WAS THE BRIGHTEST DAY?

It was on film, just before it burned out
completely and came undone. In front
of Buckingham Fountain in a line of strollers,
before my mother races toward the camera.
Then on the beach in Atlantic City,
my mother in a two-piece bathing suit
and my infant sister in a white bonnet.
The sky is white, the sand a painful yellow;
my sister squints and my mother shimmies
behind dark glasses and jet black hair.
The day lasts a fraction of a reel, two minutes
at most, and then it is dark and Christmas,
we are bundled and stamping feet at a parade.

WHEN WERE YOU LOVED WORST?

There is no bad love, just a lack
of it, and it's bad when you had love
and then it's gone, like the frogs
that sang you to sleep going extinct,
like the Norwegian maple blown down
even after you've trimmed and braced it,
like the cat that warmed your lap become
a ghost on a chair when you enter the room,
like a dry riverbed, a locust- or hail-battered crop.
I was still there but my home had turned
against me, so that I was always slightly afraid
and curled into the life raft of the couch
and looked at nothing, and tried not to think
when he talked or touched me or called my name.

WHEN WERE YOU LOVED BEST?

She loved me without question,
and ate my stories like cake.
She invited me into every space,
chose me, shared with me, shared me.

She loves me day in and day out
and over long silences still, and engages
me with joy and conversation.
Her laugh and my laugh are one.

We are two sides of a coin, that close
and every bit that far apart.
I cannot see her even as I see her.
I am filled with my need for forgiveness.

When I needed her, she rushed to my side;
without her love I think I would have died.

II

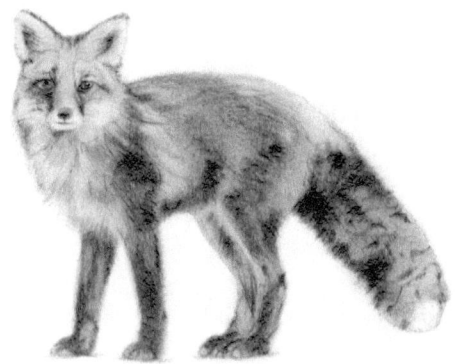

THE DEER COME CLOSE

This winter is colder longer than it has ever been.
The snow is deeper, something we thought
was over, the winters of childhood.

The deer come close to the house at night
and we see their tracks in the morning
under the white pine, even closer,
under the bedroom window, digging
and even lying down, wandering
like lost, freezing people might.

Mid-March spring doesn't come
with birdsong, but after days of rain,
the deer come in the early morning
and one lies down under the pine.
Half a dozen graze the prairie
at their leisure, stepping fetlock deep,
piercing the crusted snow.

OBSERVANCES

ON *FEBRUARY*, A PAINTING BY SOPHIA HEYMANS

The painting is carried across the field to live with you.
In it you recognize everything except the perspective.
There's nowhere you can stand to see that much,
not even on your porch, not even your roof.

No place you can see every crooked nursery tree
and your own garden and the pig barns, too,
and the pine grove, and all three houses,
and your husband's track across snow to his shop,
and there, look—someone skiing the perimeter.

You have to be a child of this farm, one who can fly
above it all and see beyond the windbreaks,
one who can hover in the cold winter sky
for all the days needed to capture it.

PRAIRIE, EARLY SPRING

Ash, smoldering white edges
and patches blacker than newly turned dirt
where the prairie was carefully burned.

> *I learn to prick the seed*
> *into the cells and barely cover.*
> *Heat's up and water pressure's down*
> *in the greenhouse with the clogged pump.*

Sand hill cranes calling in the wetlands,
settling and disappearing onto their nest.

> *I say they're ours and you laugh*
> *and say they're yours.*
> *I say they may eat in your field*
> *but they come here to sleep at night.*

Stumps where he felled the rows
of cottonwoods lining the drive.

> *Three eggs. Even*
> *the sick hen is laying. I'm huffy*
> *having to steal my own chicken's eggs.*

THE POET LECTURES US ON DRAGONFLIES

The poet in Hawaii lectures us on the death of dragonflies
and all the palm varieties he's planted on his estate.
Why does he live in Hawaii? I wonder.
It's beautiful, but imports two thirds of its food.
I imagine a line of bright container ships
and big-bellied planes stuffed to hulls and holds,
powering over miles and miles of sea.
Poets are the most selfish people I know.
It's difficult to feed, not the birds, squirrels,
or butterflies, that glean and have their season,
but our own deep hungers for beauty, song,
for pineapple and palms and dragonflies.

BOTTLE GENTIAN

"Oh, what in you can answer to this blueness?"
—D. H. LAWRENCE

This gentian, too, a torch
to guide through fall's encroaching dark,

its fork of blue flames closed
to bees and butterflies, protecting

its pollen even as it attracts
the slow, last buzzing summer drones.

Go south! Monarchs start your journey
through blue sky, over blue water,

and I will draw inward like these gentians
with their sweet lavender light

while the last fireworks of lobelia
spark in ditches,

and aster clusters poke their way
through glowing fields of goldenrod.

You, gentian, would be overlooked
in any other season, among the trees,

so closed it seems you bud
but never bloom. In September

we welcome you where we find you,
those of us who, earthbound, still seek.

DAYLIGHT SAVINGS TIME

1.

Does the spinach beneath its gauze hoop know
        it is an hour earlier than this time yesterday?
Do the scallions, exposed and pointing to the sky?
Does the four-foot kale wonder why the frost melted earlier
        than yesterday?
Do the greens in the cold frame wonder if dinner will be earlier today?
Did the garlic in its bed of straw wake up more rested today?
Did the pheasants awake hungrier?

2.

We went to bed at 11 and slept an extra hour.
When we got up, we worked an extra hour before church.
It felt too early for lunch, so we went for an hour-long walk.
It was such a nice day, we spent an extra hour putting the garden
        to bed.
There was an extra hour for the babka to rise.
I forgot to take the meat from the freezer, but it had an extra hour
        to thaw.
In the early darkness, we had an extra hour to hunker down and nap.
And at bedtime, so satisfied with how we spent the day,
we gave ourselves an extra hour to read.

THE BEAUTIFUL DEAD

1

We walked out back
to see the body of the fox
my husband shot
before it could kill
the cooped chickens
or the baby sand hill cranes
or the goslings
or the ducklings.

Even I, who withdraw
my eyes from the dead—
or no— the dying, with my fear.

This living animal, this dog
who has pranced and trotted
and stalked all small life this spring,
bright orange, unmistakable, along the edge
of woodland, wetland, and prairie.

We'd scared him off with clanging
and light and human voices
but there is no keeping a fox
away once he smells life.

2

We make good use
of binoculars to count
chicks and capture on film
beauty that comes close but not too.

But the fullness of the creatures
is only available to us,
only still, approachable,
when they are dead. Thus,
there is always grief in it.

It has always been this way—
the early field guides drawn
from collections of specimens
culled by hunters and scientists,
pinned and laid out and
rendered by Audubon
back into living landscapes.

I can count on one hand
the beautiful creatures
killed since I arrived
a dozen years ago—
the pheasant, hunted

with boys and a dog, stripped clean
of his sharp, iridescent plumage
on our kitchen counter,
field corn dug from his gullet,
a lesson, before I took the breast
warm in my hand and soaked it in wine
and made a stew in justification,
and yes, I hungered for more.

The unpitiable rabbit,
long-eared and soft, produce-
thief, mad reproducer.

But both of us still feel the stain
of the sin of the beautiful owl
whose leg was caught in a trap,
who made it just to our yard,
rattling his chains in the dark,
scaring the caged birds in our care.

None was so beautiful as he was.

The owl was mistaken for a predator,
shot blind to protect chickens
he could not have reached.
But we want to blame the trap.

The bullet killed him,
this extraordinary barn owl,
and we laid him out in the morning
and marveled at his feathers,
his wide wings, his white face,
and the tragedy, telling ourselves

he couldn't have been saved, not
one-legged as he would be. That lie.

We had mistaken prey for predator,
our only atonement a promise
never again to shoot in the dark.

And this fox, sharp-toothed
but fluffy-tailed, too, in the field.
What do we have in common
with this killer? This doesn't feel
like a win at all, to have created
or simply restored on our land
a world that brings so much life
only to take it, in glory, away.

III

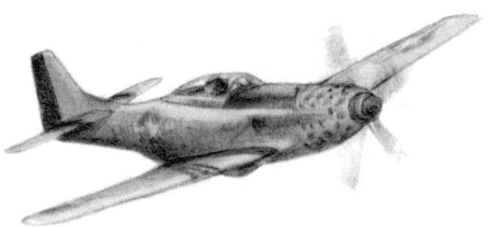

PEELS

When my mother made apple pie,
my sister and I sat at the table
and ate the long, tart peels.
She did the task with a skill
and privacy she often had.

We talked, no doubt,
saying things children say,
but I think of us as silent,
watching her wield the paring knife
and carve the apple to its core,
listening to the shearing sound,
eating the red strips like candy.

When she peeled potatoes, too,
we would sit at the table,
hungry for a salted, raw chunk,
for anything, everything, she gave.

HOW TO READ MARY OLIVER'S POETRY

FOR CONNIE EGGERS AND THE STUDENTS OF THE COLLEGE OF SAINT BENEDICT

On the college library shelves I see
all of Mary Oliver's collections
have been taken outside.

Blue Pastures was taken in the rain
and read under a pine, safe
until the wind shook down a shower.

American Primitive is so worn
its spine is like a peeled birch
whose skin was used for the canoe

where *Swan* was forgotten and sloshed
in the bottom, dug out of a pack
and dried in the sun near the chapel.

Twelve Moons was taken cross country
on skis to a monk's fish house for tea.
You can breathe in the stove smoke still.

Red Bird was hiked in a backpack
and read sitting in an Adirondack chair.
See the page smudged with mosquito, blood.

Blue Iris took a plane to lie on the beach,
where salt penetrated the pages
and sand still grinds in the spine.

A House of Light kept company
while someone crouched in weeds
awaiting the sand hill cranes.

She left a muddy fingerprint on a page
while she listened to the cranes rattling squawk
and thought even one's wild life could be elegant.

Only *Dream Work* is intact. It slept and slept
beneath pillows on the single beds
in the Women Only dorms.

Oh yes, it's true, the spine falls easily
open to the place where they learned
to embrace their simple rebellions.

MIDDLEMARCH

Isn't this the human condition?
Dorothea opens his notebooks expecting genius,
the project for which she's subjugated her life
and not insignificant intellect. George Eliot,
ungainly and plain, knowing her own mind,
creates the condition for supreme disappointment,
the house of cards collapsing, *banality,*
Mr. Casaubon less than a mere mortal, now dead,
chaining Dodo to his desk and dusty scribbles.
Worse than the loss of fortunes, we all sit
watching as the furniture is carried out,
piece by beautiful piece, packed in the wagon
and driven away, leaving us only our selves.

PARK FOREST

AFTER WILLIAM STAFFORD'S "HOME TOWN"

Peace on my twice All-American City,
on its parades and boys' baseball.

Fruitfulness like a light breeze lifting the seeds
of my first meadow, bending Queen Anne's Lace,
rustling the leaves in my first forest,
populating its food shelf and community gardens,
cultivating the backyard apples and pears
and Concord grapes along the Smith's patio.

Freedom from fear for its policemen and firemen,
for its citizens driving the orderly streets, the close quarters
of its neighborhoods, the houses stuffed with children
spilling onto bikes and skateboards and trampolines
and into double Dutch and over fences and up trees.

Light and warmth and punctual trains for the riders
of the IC casting long shadows from the platform,
preoccupied no longer with newspapers and library
thrillers but with phones and laptops and worry.
May they be wrapped in the electric and leather scent
that are caught in the chill of their coats.

Praise be for the proximity of every good thing—
the splashing mania of the city's pools,
the deep velvet-lined window seats of the library,
the cold milk and candy selection at Convenient.

Prosperity for the churches and synagogues,
their Christmas and Easter trumpets and candles,
their Good Friday processions and packed parking lots,
the Passover seder and sculpture of ploughshares.
New life in all the coming and going, all the dreaming
and pride. Let us tend to the spaces and people,
let us wave from our car windows as we drive by.

A PLANK IN REASON

IN MEMORY OF PHILIP HEYMANS

I

Geriatric Behavioral Health Ward, Litchfield, Minnesota

I am not sure why I'm here in School,
when my roommate and I are pilots—
He is flying sorties over Australia, along the coast
right now. He's an excellent pilot.
Over Africa I gave that German some trouble,
enough so he turned home in pretty bad shape.
My roommate and I are in the program together
but we don't fly together. What's his name again?
I'm telling you I'm losing names so quickly.

II

If they can get the armaments, more parish kids can go to school.
Without these deductions, it isn't going to happen.
The Japanese are concerned about the pilots they have lost.
I've never had much good to say about doctors.
These two are never going to get the deductions we need.
Don't they know we've paid into it already?
The Germans have the planes, and that big program—
what's it called again? Of course, we have Normandy.
I tried to get what I could for that school on the lake.
Most of those kids are getting what they need now.
Armaments is the word, so very accurate. What we mean
is mostly ammunition. It weighs our planes down, and the bombs.
Do you know if the war is going to end soon?

III

If we can win this tournament, St. Mary's can go all the way.
They're good kids, but not a lot of talent there.
If your brothers could come, that would help.
I've never met such mouthy kids. Even the ladies,
serving the food, working the games, such language.
And they don't care much about your privacy either.
I'm telling you the ethics, I thought this place was better,
it's really gone downhill since I was a student.

Have you heard anything? Is anyone talking about it?
What are they saying? Is it known as a Catholic place?

When this year's meetings are over—
Don't they know I need to be there?
I could actually do some good if they'd let me go—
my roommate and I are flying to Brillion,
I'm desperate to get units from the new line;
I can't sell them if I don't have them.
Please keep an eye open for the parts they're sending
and if you can get a hold of any of the new machines,
you have my permission to go ahead. Sign for them.

Who authorized this whole thing?

IV

Mother of Mercy Senior Living, Albany, Minnesota

I want to see my wife.
Why hasn't my wife visited me
for at least three days?
Would you go across the street
and check on my wife, and call me back?

My mother was worried this morning.
I told her I'd check in later today.
She'll be wondering where I am.

My dad needed me to do something
with him. He'll be expecting me.
When can I get out of here?
I need to get over there.
Has anyone checked on mother and dad?
Do you know how they're doing?
They'll be wondering where I am.

Where is my wife now? Does she know
I'm here? Why hasn't she been to visit?

At this point I don't need the car keys.
You don't have to take me there.
I can hitchhike. I've done it plenty of times.
This thumb will get me home.

V

If we leave right now we can be home by dinner.
Home with my wife—I have business
to take care of down there,
the taxes to be paid, business, deals.
We can just go for one day and then come back.
My bags are packed, I'm ready to go.
I talked to her on the phone yesterday,
and I could hear her voice break.

I built that house? Are you kidding me?
I don't remember any of that. See, Betty,
I've never had a good memory. I've always got along
not remembering those things.

Isn't it strange? I can remember so clearly
that plane that went down in Sleepy Eye Lake—
the landing gear was down, but it was a sea plane,
and it flipped over. My dad and I rowed out.
I can see it, I can hear it, so clearly to this day.

And my first day of school, when I came home
and cried because I still couldn't read,
school hadn't worked for me at all.
How can I remember that, and the Notre Dame score
last week, and not remember building that house
or who lives there, and who they are to me?

This room keeps following me around.
No matter where I go, when I come back
it's always this room. In Sleepy Eye
or in Avon or Albany, anywhere they take me

this room is there. One weekend I was
in Morris, and the room was just the same.
I touched everything to make sure it was real.
Not just the television—the chair, the bed,
everything was exactly like this room here.
We have to do something about this room.
It just keeps following me. I just keep ending up here.

IV

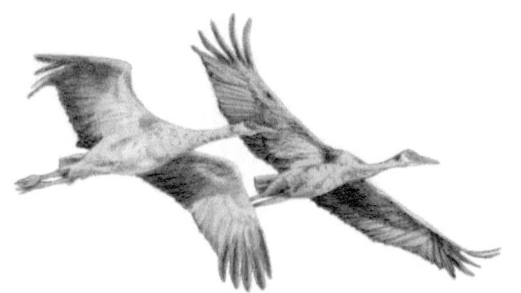

THE FIRST MORNING

The first morning I wake up
with cancer, the neighbor's dog
is barking and barking,
something she has never done before.

WAYS TO PRAY FOR HEALING

"The prayers of all good people are good."
—WILLA CATHER, *MY ANTONIA*

There are many people praying
(even Congregationalists in Connecticut)

and a candle lit before the Madonna and Child,
and prayer chains with my name on them

and Novenas being said in Rome, in Lourdes,
and others sitting in silence and holding me there.

Candles everywhere, and a lantern in the woods,
and intercessions to St. Peregrine, and a children's choir,

and so many people "holding good thoughts"
and "sending positive, healing energy."

Then this question comes in over the web:
"Is there an image you'd like me to carry for you?"

It makes one think, that question.

I know that I am imagining the cancer
in the lining of my ovaries, as mold,

the kind that gets on shower walls
(I've never been much of a housekeeper),

or like the inside of a kiwi, based on a photo
I saw of cancer cells swimming under a microscope

and the chemo as this powerful cleanser, on the order
of Drano, or a product charged with scrubbing bubbles,

(which no one wants to have in their bloodstream,
but you have to admit it does a specific job very well)

poured via port into my jugular vein to wash out
all that residue, that slime of cancer, wherever it is.

So that my lungs can clear of fluid, and my ovary walls
will show no more bright spots on the PET scan.

But that's not what this person means.

OK then, how about my soon-to-be bald head
and my smile, (leave the eyebrows intact, please).

An elderly woman in the grocery said to me last year:
"How lucky—you will always have your dimples."

But that's not what she means. She means some totem
to carry in her pocket that would say "healing," or "journey,"

and all I can think of is a jade turtle, or a soapstone frog,
or an ivory heron, or a well-sanded wood swan.

Or the paths in our prairie after a burn,
or five chickens coming around the side of the house,
or the cry of the sand hill cranes, or pea sprouts, or a radish seed.

Or carry a smooth pebble in your mouth,
or a shell worn to abalone shimmer by the sea,
and taste the salt, or I mean, the pearl.

I don't know at all what image she should carry.
I don't know what God looks like, just that God is everywhere.

FREEZE AND THAW

They enter the new world naked,
cold, uncertain of all
save that they enter. All about them
the cold, familiar wind—

FROM "SPRING AND ALL" BY WILLIAM CARLOS WILLIAMS

The maples are hung with IV bags.
Too many patients, two thousand,
staked on the brown hills. The woods are ill.

At the clinic, 36 rooms for infusions,
each the same: a patient, a nurse, an IV.
We look metallic. We look poisoned.

I'm thinking of poetry—Williams
on his way to the contagion hospital,
Eliot's sky etherized on a table.

Am I to become a Modernist now?
Eschewing nature, or feeling cold
instead of the stirrings of spring?

Maple syrup requires thaw by day
and freeze each night to make
the sap run. Usually it is enlivening,

but now, too much intrusion,
too much plastic and something stolen,
something scarred, despite custom-made spiles.

Gunmetal sky. Ironwood trees. Copper marsh.
I trudge instead of walk and tire easily.
All I taste is metal. Uncertain of all.

PETTING THE RAY

How do you understand
a stomach ache? That cauldron
of acids into which you've poured
ingredients odder than eye of newt
rejects what it cannot dissolve.
That pink pouch, that engine of energy,
breaking down the spaghetti and meatball,
sending protein here and carbs
(What's a carb?) there, and eliminating
the rest—down to the bowels, the bowels!
That coiled snake, gorging on our bad choices,
crushing waste like a stack of discarded cars.
When the surgeon talked about stripping
the bowel lining, I thought of a car
and wondered what lubricant
I could feed myself—castor oil?
The liver, dense triangle straddling
whatever organ it straddles,
darkest red and meaty rich,
encased in a tight web of blood vessels.
In the initial scan, glowing with disease,
there was a bright slug sitting on it.
(We salted it.)

The most reassuring
and the most disturbing
thing the surgeon said
is that she slid her hand
under my ribs into inoperable
space, and felt my lung.

Like petting the rays at the aquarium
or riding a dolphin, she touched
what had been inviolable, beyond
reach, that granite slab, that sedum bloom,
and it was smooth, no stubby nodules,
no pink polyps, no whorled white tumors,
nothing but lung resting in its slip of lining,
clear, all clear, we hope beyond hope, clear.

AT FIFTY-FOUR, THE AGE I WAS PREDICTED TO DIE

I have lived exactly twice as long
as Jimi Hendrix, Janice Joplin, Curt Cobain,
and also Jim Morrison and Amy Winehouse.

I have heard so much music
in the last twenty-seven years,
and seen so much good art
and films that amazed me with their stories.

I have had two marriages and so many friends,
lived in Chicago, Reno, and California,
before settling on the prairie in Minnesota.
I bought and sold two lovely homes.

I camped high in the Sierras and swam
in alpine lakes with granite bottoms,
cool and clear and deep and unpeopled.
I spent considerable time
committing them to memory, because I knew
I would need them someday close at hand.
Think of all the people who haven't seen them.

I was a teacher, an editor, told the stories
of a large community of nuns—
stood outside the chapel door waiting
for the announcement of a new prioress,
wrote the press release—it was as exciting
as watching for smoke at the Vatican.

I have grown food, I grow food still!
What a thing to learn to do, and to have space
and be able to turn the soil and know
the times to plant different crops
and how far apart to space them
and to water and weed and harvest
and preserve and open the jars in winter!

I have been a poet and a writer
in the company of other poets and artists
and famous novelists, photographers,
and even composers of operas!
So when I am feeling low
about what I have lost
and what I still have to lose,
at limitations and missed opportunities,
I don't have to look far at all
to see all I've gained, savored,
the utter lack of tragedy,
truly, the joy, of going into the world
and coming home, and being home.

FRANKINCENSE

BEFORE PALM SUNDAY, RECURRENCE AFTER TWO-YEAR REMISSION

I smell like church.
I wake to the scent of the censor
swinging, the smoke rising.

Last night, anxious over the scan
I dotted the oil on my chest,
willing it into my lungs,

and another necklace
on my abdomen, place of origin,
in case anything still lives there.

Rubbing it into my skin,
the essential oil scented my fingers
which scented my pillows.

Exotic fragrance of far away,
the tiny rocks brought by the kings,
this oil credited for healing

my specific disease. This morning,
despite the talisman, the news is bad,
not what I wanted, and I am afraid.

I smell like cancer.
I step through a veil of normality
into today's Cancerland.

I enter the world of slow-motion dying,
cycles of treatment and recurrence.
On Sunday I will start to travel

to Jerusalem, to Calvary,
with the baby visited by kings,
born to die for our sins.

HEALING

Always I have considered *healing*
and believed

>   we get it wrong.

In church, we laid on our hands,
but the woman healed of a brain tumor
eventually died of a brain tumor.

How the people pressed on Jesus
as he walked on the road,

touched his cloak,
lowered a lame man through the roof,
sent their servants to beg his power,

and again and again he said
it wasn't him at all, but faith.

He used these opportunities
to talk about the kingdom of God
and eyes that could see
and ears that could hear.

mud, cloak, litter

Only Lazarus, when Jesus arrived late,
and so then, and only then,
his love reached beyond the grave
and brought the man from death

to life, ordinary, in a body, in a family,
with more years of suffering and joy.

THIS WEATHER

This weather is for A.
whose time is we don't know
how long or short or springs
or summers or falls how many.

This weather is for A.
anxious to get back
to her island which is north
and reached by ferry
we don't know how close
or far or how many more times.

This weather is for A.,
these frogs and the chives
and grass and maple sap
and thaw by day and freeze
and we don't know how warm
or long or cold or back and forth.

This weather is for A.
to get to her island
and eat berries with syrup
for long and summer long.

WAITING FOR THE BIOPSY RESULTS

No word as of 5 pm Friday
so the clock stops
until Monday at 8 am

and nothing can be done
but wait. No matter,
I tell myself, since

I have been given
two possibilities,
a bad cancer or worse one.

Though Friday night I dream
I am handed a report that reads:
benign. A nurse repeats: *benign*.

It wakes me up, and I wonder
how long it has been
since I even thought the word

     benign

It is not even
in my vocabulary.
My eyes fly open and I laugh.

Still, there can be
no next steps,
no matter how ready I am

until the pathologist
tightens the focus
on the microscope slide

and on the numbers
and writes and posts
the report.

I know a pathologist.
He told me what my blood cells
enhanced by medication look like:

larger and slipperier
than regular ones, and more,
which is the point.

I want to call him up,
and tell him to get to my lab
and call me right away.

Instead I walk in the cold,
take naps, somehow get
to Monday 8 am, and wait.

THE RESULTS

When the results ping my phone
I pull to the side of the road.
There is the word from my dream:
benign
benign, benign, benign, I want
to inscribe pink helium balloons
and float them to my ceiling,
and fill a room with their buoyancy.
    Benign, benign, benign.
In the months ahead I find I'm done
still with the black shoe of breasts,
benign just means no new cancer to fight,
that coal lump my familiar cancer.

WHILE I WAS GONE

AN ADVENT POEM, IN REMISSION

While I was gone the twins at church grew
from girls to young women, recognizable
by their waterfalls of hair still tucked into a pew.

While I was in treatment the city tore up
the straight road to my door
and made a curved tract for six houses.

At my bedroom window I watched
crops planted, crops growing,
the bright lights of harvesters at night.

From the screen porch I saw small, red birds
and hopping goldfinches and bandit-eyed
orioles, all in pairs, and one woodpecker.

The light grew longer day by day,
rain fell on the solstice,
and the days grew shorter again.

See the twins take wrapped gifts
to put under the tree,
on the altar near the nativity.

I am here to see the waterfalls of hair
and the same priest processing
and hear the same old story, the annual promise.

EARLIEST SPRING

If you ask my favorite season
I will always say fall.
Who can resist the copper
bright blue clarity of it?

Who can fail but delight
in harvest abundance,
sated, straw-colored animals
and pregnant moons?

Here in Minnesota,
spring is only a calculation
of freeze and thaw splitting
the distance from summer.

When is the last snow?
Don't plant too early.
Parrying jabs and crosses,
potholes and mud.

But the earliest spring
fulfills promises
we should not overlook:
more life (not always a given).

It comes with light
that sings to seeds
and stirs the chickens
to lay again.

FERTILITY

ON *MAY,* A PAINTING BY SOPHIA HEYMANS

From the shape of the patch I say
it is a wetland, round and marshy
and verdant at the edges,
floppy stands of last year's sedge
scored like fireworks into the canvas.

From the trees I say it aspires
to be an oak savannah,
rooted and long-standing,
wise and showing off its age,
upper branches a roost for hawks
though not quite yet.

The border tells a different story:
rows upon cultivated rows,
brown and clean and waiting
for the dark sky to drop its rain,
and reaching in, bottom right,
a row of brighter green new leaves.

But it is the laundry that tells me
about the freshness of the sky
and the warmth of the sun,
and it is the curve of her belly
that tells me about this ripe season
and all the life that is to come.

LATE MAY, LATE AFTERNOON

AFTER JANE KENYON'S "LET EVENING COME"

Let the light of late afternoon
call the chickens back to the run
but not yet to the coop to roost.

Let the mower crank and roar
as the man rushes to fit in
one more chore before dinner.

Let the warm shovel handle
and the blade sunk in the bed
retire upright in the garden.

Let the swallows dip and weave
to catch the bugs hovering
as heat and breeze both die

and let the pond go to glass,
tiny ripples and shadows
making the scene a woodcut,

and let the canoe paddle dip
and trail a necklace of drops
onto the bureau mirror of lake.

Let the pheasant clear its throat
and ticks burrow into the blood
and the warblers warble.

Days grow longer and longer
even as they are fewer, and still—
the light calls us to lift ourselves

like a sheet unclipped from the line
lofted, rising high over the bed,
releasing its scent as it drifts down.

I AM NOT DONE

Eighty-five years old, Stanley Kunitz told us
in a loud, sure, vibrating voice:
Live in the layers, not on the litter.

It was all of a piece, learning to embrace
uncertainty, complexity, rejecting the surface,
rejecting certainty, burrowing down.

He heard it from a "nimbus-clouded voice"
and claimed he could not decipher its meaning.
Yet I still shout this line, *Live in the layers!*

in the bathroom mirror, on walks,
in the voice of the esteemed elder poet I saw
thirty years ago, someone else's dream.

Such was the prophecy of those times,
our sense that poetry could hold experience
and also the pronouncements of mystics.

I almost lost myself in those days,
though some principle of being abides,
which has only grown more pronounced.

These days my dreams are full of confusion,
carrying words that have no meaning, only
to drop the needless burdens as the scene unfolds.

It is the litter, I suppose, striving in the dream
to grasp or earn or win a magic token
that I can see is of no help at all.

And only now, listening online,
the old man reads his poem, and I see
it doesn't end in the layers or the litter.

It ends with this, the line I need most,
as I wait for what comes next:
I am not done with my changes.

ACKNOWLEDGEMENTS

These poems were written over the course of eighteen years, and the sonnets in Section I include the oldest poems and also the very newest. Writing poetry has always been an examen/examination of the stuff of my life, making sense of and ordering "the story." My last book, *H is for Harry* (2016) was published the month after I began treatment for stage IV ovarian cancer. It looks back to my formation as a poet, and looks back to make sense of a failed marriage, and moves into the early days on the prairie and into a new, successful marriage.

This book also looks back to my formation as a poet, and into years dealing with other kinds of loss, including the deaths of my in-laws. Years of life, productive and challenging, life and dying and death on the prairie. Art and beauty and love on the prairie. Always moving forward in life even as, for the last eight years, we've staved off dying.

For their work reading and organizing and responding to the poems and this manuscript, I am grateful to my Stegner colleagues Yvonne C. Murphy and Martha Greenwald, my Sarah Lawrence colleague April Lindner, Collegeville Institute friend Tom Montgomery Fate, and dear friend Emily Wilmer, who also named the book. I am also deeply grateful to Oliver Smith, whom I've known since Atlanta in 1987, whose friendship was formative for me and who generously did the interior drawings for the collection.

For loving me best, I am ever grateful to my niece Dale, my sister Kathy, and my husband Steve.

www.ingramcontent.com/pod-product-compliance
Lightning Source LLC
Chambersburg PA
CBHW020329290526
45785CB00007B/2975